COVID-19 LOCI OF INFECTION

COVID-19 LOCI OF INFECTION

transport pathways and mechanisms

Michael M Nikoletseas

Contents

Contents

Preface

This book was written during the first few weeks of the COVID-19 pandemic.

As the first clinical reports emerged, it became clear that this disease did not fit known existing schemata, in particular, the sudden dramatic pulmonary component.

In the belief that detailed neuroanatomic knowledge may help clinicians understand better the spread and progression of this disease and thus devise more efficient preventive as well as therapeutic interventions, I wrote this book.

Dr. Michael M Nikoletseas
Medical anatomist

April 30, 2020

Introduction

Molecular interventions in the treatment of COVID-19 and other viral diseases are indisputably powerful. However, we should not lose sight of the need for multilevel studies which offer complementary knowledge that may not be constrained by the strict specificity of molecular approaches. The best strategy is to prevent the virus from entering the body or effecting a decrease in the rate and extent of infection.

Case studies as well as informal reports coming from physicians treating COVID-19 paint a picture of an atypical respiratory disease with an erratic, unpredictable progression. This may be an indication that a non-systemic contribution plays a more important role than it has so far been admitted. I propose a pseudo-quantal contribution to the progression of this disease by various points of entry, pathways and mechanisms as exemplified in the nervous system. A tentative proposition emerges that COVID-19 is partly a nervous system disease [1].

Loci and pathways of transmission of the virus may be neural or non-neural. Any surface of the body, cutaneous, epithelial or mucous may provide favorable ground for the virus to attach and invade deeper tissues and organs. Mouth, nose, eyes, ears, genitals, anus are loci for which the probability of incipient infections is greater. Local infections may become systemic. To this list less apparent loci must be added, for example *emissary veins* and trauma. In time the virus may gain access to the nervous system, vascular pathways and the lymphatic system.

PART A

Non-neural transmission

Any part of the body is a potential site of viral infection and further transmission to other parts, however the probability of its developing into a serious disease is not the same for all body locations. A gross classification of possible loci of infection is *non-neural* (mouth, nose, eyes, ears) and *neural* (cutaneous and epithelial nerve endings and, more significantly, cranial nerves).

The Mouth

Entry of the virus through the mouth is highly probable on account of its frontal location and its function in social and biological acts. From the buccal cavity it may spread to the pharynx, nasopharynx, and via the larynx and the esophagus to the lungs and the digestive system respectfully. Factors like pH and local chemistry may inhibit or destroy the virus.

Of exceptional significance is the potential transmission from the buccal to the nasal cavity and the middle ear via the *Eustachian tube*. Infection in the middle ear may further spread to the inner ear via the *oval* and *round windows* and thence to the cerebrospinal fluid (CSF) intracranially. Additionally, from the middle ear, the virus may reach the brainstem via axonal transport im the *trigeminal nerve* (*tensor tymapni* muscle), the *facial nerve* (*stapedius* muscle), and *chorda tympani*.

{ 2 }

The Nose

The nasal cavity is perhaps the most important locus in contacting the virus as well as in the further propagation and severity of subsequent infection. In the absence of consumed foodstuffs and liquids, enzymes and saliva, the nasal cavity may be an ideal environment for contact, survival, multiplication and further propagation.

The nasal cavity communicates with the *frontal, parietal, and sphenoidal sinuses* via small openings, ostia. Infections of the sinuses may be part of the pseudo-quantal contribution to the progression of the COVID-19 disease as they may empty at irregular intervals into the nasal cavity and thence into the nasopharynx and subsequently reach the lungs. It is possible that the infection spreads directly into the cranial cavity. *Sphenoidal sinus* infection has been linked to cranial nerve transient abnormalities probably because of spread of infection into the *cavernous sinus*. These cranial nerves may transmit the virus to their respective nuclei in the brainstem.

In certain circumstances, nasal infections may be transmitted intracranially through the many *foramina* of the *cribriform plate*. A similar route for direct transmission of the virus intracranially is through *emissary veins* (*parietal, styloid, posterior cranial fossa*) which, however are not always present.

Retropharyngeal space

Related to nasopharynx is the possible spread of infection to the *retropharyngeal* and *danger spaces* and thence to the *mediastinum*. Retropharyngeal infections are known to be associated with upper respiratory infections, although the possibility of pulmonary disease from mediastinal infections exists. A recent study [2] reported that 19.7% of Covid-19 patients in Wuhan China suffered cardiac injury which in turn was a risk factor contributing to death. This finding has raised vivid interest in the medical community worldwide. The mechanism and details of the association of cardiac injury and Covid-19 are not known. In addition to autonomic factors, the involvement of the retropharyngeal space may play a role.

The retropharyngeal space is potential space between the *alar fascia* and *buccopharyngeal fascia* in the cervical area continuing as *danger space* into the posterior *mediastimum* as far as the diaphragm. Known long before imaging, it is distinguishable on CT or MRI in case of fluid accumulation as a result of infection. Such infection may spread to the carotid sheath (*carotid artery, jugular vein, glossopharyngeal, vagus, spinal accessory cranial nerves*) superiorly, and inferiorly via the danger space to the posterior mediastinum as far as the diaphragm, thus potentially affecting the heart. Bacterial and viral retropharyngeal infections are known to occur in children but also adults. There is an association between viral upper-respiratory infections and retropharyngeal infections. It is also known that acute myocardial infarction can be precipitated by acute respiratory infections. As in the case of Covid-19 patients, retropharyngeal infections occur more frequently in males. It is worth investigating a possible association between retropharyngeal infections and Covid-19.

{ 4 }

The Eye

The eye is one of the three major frontal openings of the head, the other two being the mouth and the nose. The other major opening of the head is the ear on the lateral surface. It is noteworthy that the eye has not been given the same weight as a possible entry of viruses as the mouth and nose; masks covering the mouth and nose, but not glasses, figure prominently in prophylactic measures instituted by such health agencies as the World Health Organization (WHO) and the US Center for Disease Control (CDC). The ear has been totally ignored.

Viral infection of the the cornea may be transmitted to midbrain nuclei via axonal transport in the trigeminal nerve. Infections in the orbit may be transmitted to the brainstem nuclei of the motor nerves (CNIII, CNIV, CNVI) that innervate the extraocular muscles,

Parasymphathetic efferent fibers to the *constrictor pupilae* and the *ciliary muscle* may transmit viral infections to the brainstem (*Edinger-Westphal nucleus*).

Viral infection of the eyebulb or the orbit may spread to

the *lacrimal gland* and thence to the *pterygopalatine ganglion* where they synapse with the preganglionic parasympathetic fibers of the *lacrimatory nucleus* of the facial nerve in the pons (*nervus untermedius*-facial nerve-*greater petrosal* nerve-*deep petrosal* nerve-*nerve of the pterygoid canal*- *pterygopalatine ganglion*-*zygomatic* and *zygomaticotemporal* nerves-lacrimal branch of the the ophthalmic division of the trigeminal nerve-lacrimal gland).

Axonal transport of virus from the *lacrimal gland*, although possible, would be minimal in because of the intervening synapse in the *pterygopalatien ganglion* and the very small diameter of the *greater petrosal nerve*.

Viral infection of the eye or the lacrimal gland may be transmitted to the nasal cavity in tears via the *lacrimal duct*.

Infection of the retina would lead to virus transmission via *anterograde axonal transport* in the ganglion cells of CNII to the *lateral geniculate nucleus* of the thalamus and thence to the *occipital* cortex bilaterally, and the *superior colliculus*.

The Ear

In reviewing experimental work on human coronaviruses (HCoV) and other neuroinvasive viruses as well as case studies of COVID-19 patients, it becomes apparent that entry of the virus occurs mainly via the mouth and nose. Early in the covid-19 pandemic I alerted the health agencies of another entry gate of the virus, that of the ear. Given that the tympanic membrane is patent not only in cases of genetic patency or perforation due to trauma, but also via active and passive transport, the route external acoustic meatus, middle ear, Eustachian tube, nasopharynx, larynx, trachea, lungs is a direct path for the virus to the interior of the lungs. In these early reports I also pointed out a potentially important path

for the virus to the mediastinum and thus the heart and the outer surface of the lungs, that of the retropharyngeal, danger space. Cardiac injury was observed in covid-19 patients in the Wuhan original studies and subsequently elsewhere. The retropharyngeal route may explain the observed cardiac injury and its so-far characterization as entailing oddities.

PART B

Neural transmission

An optimal therapeutic method for respiratory diseases must be based on multi-level knowledge. Given that respiration is a motor response, it is necessary that coronavirus research on all aspects of the central as well as peripheral nervous system (neuroanatimical neurophysiological, neurohormonal and neurochemical) be given high priority. Until studies on the new coronavirus are conducted, we rely on studies on other viruses.

The respiratory center consists of nerve cell nuclei in the central nervous system (CNS), namely brainstem (*pons* and *medulla oblongata*). Although the most dramatic and most definitive event in the COVID-19 disease is difficulty to breathe, disproportionately less attention has been paid to the neural components of the disease. In the present book I review the basic anatomy of the nervous circuitry of respiration as well the possible loci of virus entry to the CNS along cranial nerves.

The motor response of respiration is effected by neuronal

assemblies (nuclei) in the brainstem (*pons* and *medulla oblongata*) as well as *autonomic* (*sympathetic* and *parasympathetic*) and *branchial* centers. It is important to keep in mind that respiration is not an *autonomic* response. The efferent output of the brainstem centers to the diaphragm via the *phrenic nerve* is not autonomic. The diaphragm is not smooth muscle, it is skeletal. Autonomic control of respiration occurs on the intrinsic muscles of the lungs. In this sketchy description I omit the subtle cardiovascular-pulmonary regulatory responses as well as the role of chemoreptors. Consideration of the *branchial* nervous system as such is perhaps of little clinical significance.

It is knowledge of these facts that guide interventions of the anesthesiologist and the emergency medicine physician. In the treatment of COVID-19 disease we must not confine our interventions to principally immunological or emergency protocol, but should also lay out the spatiotemporal progression of the infection in the nervous system.

In this report I point out the importance of neuroanatomical, neurophysiologic facts in critical events in COVID-19 disease. Axonal retrograde and anterograde transport in viral infections have been documented. Knowledge of the spatial and temporal parameters may be valuable in devising interventions that may block the spread of the virus or at least lessen the magnitude of its impact in time. The temporal course of virus transport in neurons depends on distance and axonal characteristics and takes place in a few days. Invasion of the CNS in the case of respiratory viruses is very rapid, given the short distance from olfactory nerve cells in the upper part of the nasal cavity to the *olfactory bulbs*, and hence, the short distance to the base of the brain, *piriform cortex*, *diencephalon* and farther, the brainstem. A speculative account of the effects of CNS infection on observed pathology would include thermoregulation (diencephalon), stress and mineralcorticoid hormone disturbances (hypothalamus-neurohypophysis) as well as pituitary peptides.

Subsequent invasion of the respiratory centers would affect respiration. A generalized infection of brainstem nuclei would profoundly disrupt vital functions as well as general efferent and afferent signals. Knowledge of the spatial and temporal map as outlined here can serve as the basis for a host of interventions, pharmacological and other. For example, blocking or retarding the rate of viral invasion of the CNS may be effected at the level of the nasal epithelium, *cribriform plate* or olfactory bulb. We may take advantage of the fact that olfactory nerve cells that reside in the nasal epithelium regenerate, and selectively inactivate or destroy them. Similarly we may block viral neuropropagation by interfering with olfactory bulb afferents. For example, destruction of nerve cells in the olfactory bulbs by zinc sulfate.

Pulmonary disease is the most grave culmination of COVID-19 infection. In treating pulmonary disease disproportionately less emphasis has been given to the fact that respiration is a motor response in direct control of CNS motor centers.

All twelve cranial nerves are possible routes of viral transmission to the CNS. Given that the respiration centers reside in the brainstem (pons, medulla oblongata), the cranial nerves whose nuclei are in the brainstem are of special significance in COVID-19 disease.

CNI olfactory nerve

The cell bodies of the olfactory nerve reside in the upper part of the nasal cavity and therefore are exposed to airborne viruses that cause respiratory infections. Axons of olfactory cells form fascicles that enter the cranial cavity through foramina of the *cribriform plate* and synapse on the olfactory bulbs. Olfactory information is thence relayed to the olfactory cortical centers.

The fact that CNI does not have a nucleus in the brainstem minimizes its importance in acute viral respiratory disease. However, animal studies [3] have shown that viral infection of the nasal epithelium is transported via axonal transport of CNI to the olfactory bulb and in about five days it reaches the brainstem.

Several species of viruses that enter the CNS via the olfactory nerve have been reported: *influenza A virus, herpesviruses, poliovirus, paramyxoviruses, vesicular stomatitis virus, rabies virus, parainfluenza virus, adenoviruses, Japanese encephalitis virus, West Nile*

virus, chikungunya virus, La Crosse virus, mouse hepatitis virus, and *bunyaviruses* [4]. The mechanism may be diffusion or axonal transport. Spread within the CNS may involve trans-synaptic transport and diffusion-like process.

CNII optic nerve

The optic nerve is formed by axons of the *ganglion cells* whose cell bodies reside in the retina. Fibers of the optic nerve reach the *lateral geniculate ganglion* (LGN) of the thalamus where they synapse, some travel to the midbrain and synapse on the *pretectal nucleus* and the *superior colliculus,* and others synapse on the *suprachiasmatic nucleus* (SCN) of the hypothalamus. Fibers from LGN synapse on the visual areas of the occipital lobe of the brain,

Viral infections of the optic nerve [5] may spread to its synaptic locations, including the brainstem thus contributing to respiratory disease.

{ 8 }

CNIII oculomotor nerve

The *oculomotor nerve* innervates the following extraocular muscles that control eye movements for the purpose of fixating on an object: *superior rectus muscle, medial rectus muscle, inferior rectus muscle, inferior oblique muscle*. It also innervates *levator palpebrae superioris muscle* that elevates the upper eye lid. The nucleus of CNIII (*oculomotor nucleus*) is located in the midbrain at the level of the *superior colliculus*. Adjacent to it is the *accessory parasympathetic nucleus (Edinger-Westphal nucleus)* the fibers of which travel with CNIII to the orbit and innervate the *sphincter pupillae,* stimulation of which triggers *miosis,* and the *ciliary muscles* which, when activated change the curvature of the eye bulb.

Viral infection of the eye bulb, the orbit, or the cavernous sinus would spread to the midbrain via retrograde axonal transport in CNIII.

Involvement of CNIII in COVID-19 disease has been reported [6]

CNIV trochlear nerve

The *trochlear nerve* innervates one of the extraocular muscles, the *superior oblique*. It has the smallest diameter of all cranial nerves and is the only cranial nerve that exits the brainstem on the dorsal surface ot the brainstem caudal to the *inferior colliculus*, The nucleus of CNIV resides in the midbrain.

Viral infections of CNIV are rare although isolated fourth-nerve palsies of viral causes have been reported [7] Retrograde axonal transport in CNIV is possible from viral infections in the orbit or the cavernous sinus, the magnitude of which would be very small due to its minuscule axonal diameter. Efferent connections to the trochlear nucleus as well as local diffusion-like processes may carry viruses to this locus.

CNV trigeminal nerve

The *trigeminal nerve* has three divisions (roots) *ophthalmic* (V1), *maxillary* (V2), and *mandibular* (V3). V1 and V2 are sensory to the eye, and maxilla and nasal cavity respectively, while V3 is motor to the muscles of mastication and sensory to the mandibular area. The taste fibers that synapse on taste buds in the anterior two-thiirds of the tongue are fibers of the *chorda tympani* and do not belong to the trigeminal nerve; they simply take a ride with the *lingual* branch of V3 on their way to the tongue (taste) and parasympathetic ganglia for salivation,

Possibility for axonal transport of virus in the trigeminal exists. V1 is an easy route since it innervates the cornea of the eye, one of the four major openings of the head through which the virus may enter the body. Viral infection of the nasal cavity and the sinuses can gain access to the main trigeminal sensory nucleus in the brainstem (midpons) or the spinal trigeminal nucleus via axonal transport of V2. Axonal transport in V3 can occur via mandibular gums and be transmitted to the motor or the sensory nucleus. It is less likely that infection can occur via the muscles of mastication. The same holds for the fibers of the *mesencephalic nucleus* of V which carries proprioceptive information from these muscles. However, the possibility of viral axonal transport from the tensor muscles (*tensor veli palatini* and *tenor tympani*) does exist.

Infection of the *external acoustic meatus*, one of the four major opening of the head, can be transmitted to the brainstem via *trigeminal, glossopharyngeal, facial,* and *vagus nerves* [8]

CNV infections by neurotropic viruses, notably Herpesviruses are well known in clinical practice [9].

CNVI abducens nerve

CNVI innervates the *lateral rectus muscle*, one of the extraocular muscles that move the eyebulb. It also sends some fibers to the *medial rectus* thus allowing for conjugate movements of the eyebulb. The cell bodies of this nerve reside in the abducens nucleus in the dorsal pons. Viral axonal transport may occur either from infections in the orbit or the cavernous sinus through which CNVI passes along with the trochlear nerve, the oculomotor nerve, and the first branch of the trigeminal nerve (V1). Infection of the cavernous sinus may occur either from the *angular vein* (an *emissary vein* off the facial vein) or from the sphenoidal sinus.

Viral infection of CNVI have been reported [10, 11].

CNVII facial nerve

The *facial nerve* consists of efferent fibers that originate in the *facial nucleus* and innervate the following muscles:: *muscles of facial expression, stylohyoid muscle, platysma, posterior belly of digastric, stapedius, occipitofrontalis*. The facial nerve, along with V, IX, X, and XI carry efferent fibers of the *branchial* nervous system (*special visceral efferent (SVE)*, the origin of which can be traced in the respiratory apparatus of fishes. Although the branchial nervous system is more often than not classified as somatic motor, it may prove profitable to keep the discrimination live in clinical practice of respiratory conditions. The branchial motor system is characterized by exquisite sensitivity and low thresholds reactivity to environmental stimulation [12]. In primates this correlates with the low threshold and subtlety of facial expression, and vocalization.

The facial nucleus is located in the caudal pons and receives efferent fibers from the spinal trigeminal nucleus (corneal blink and other trigeminofacial reflexes), the *supe-*

rior olivary complex (stapedius reflex), and corticofugal input. Viral infections on the face or any of the innervated muscles may reach the pons via retrograde axonal transport. It is possible that viral infections in the buccal cavity may spread in the parotid salivary glands and infect the facial nerve which is embedded in them.

The facial nerve also carries (at some point of its course) somatosensory fibers from the *pinna* (*spinal trigeminal nucleus*), gustatory afferents from the tongue and palate (*solitary nucleus*), and visceral efferents of *nervus intermedius* (*superior salivatory nucleus*). Viral infections of the target structures of these fibers may reach their respective nuclei via axonal transport.

Infection of CNVII by neurotropic viruses are frequent [9]. Experimental studies reported infections of the nerve and *geniculate ganglion* after injections of human viruses in distal sites [13].

{ 13 }

CNVIII
vestibulocochlear
nerve

Involvement of the *vestibulocochlear nerve* in COVID-19 disease would occur in the event of viral infection in the middle ear and subsequent spread of the virus in the cochlea. From the cochlea the virus may reach the *vestibular nuclei* in the brainstem through axonal transport.

CNVIII neuritis may be caused by a variety of viruses and conditions [14].

Labyrinthitis often follows upper respiratory viral infections. A possible path of transmission is the *Eustachian tube–* middle ear and subsequent spread to the vestibule of the inner ear via the *oval window (vestibular window)*. Infection of the inner ear may spread to the *CSF* via the *cochlear canaliculus* and *endolymphatic duct,* in which case infection would instantly spread instantly to the entire nervous system, brain and spinal cord.

CNIX glossopharyngeal nerve

The involvement of CNIX in COVID-19 disease is apparent in view of the persistent dry cough and throat pain in the early stages of the disease, as this nerve provides sensory innervation of the pharynx. It is the afferent limb of the reflex arc of the *gag reflex*, the motor limb being CNX, *vagus nerve*. The reported loss of taste may also involve CNIX as it innervates the posterior one-third of the tongue.

What has not been paid attention to is the potential role of CNIX in the later, more dramatic stages of the disease. Following the infection of the pharynx, *soft palate*, or *Eustachian tube*, the virus may reach the nucleus of the glossopharyngeal nerve, *nucleus solitarius*, in the medulla by retrograde axonal transport.

In addition to being the home of all visceral afferents, nucleus solitarius is involved in regulation via projections to cardiac, respiratory and gastrointestinal regulatory centers.

Once in the brainstem, the virus may spread to the adjacent medullary and possibly pontine centers of respiration and cause varying degrees of dyspnea. Protracted problems in breathing may not be simply signs of neural damage but may also be on the causal side of the serious pulmonary disease that ensues in the last stages of COVID-19.

CNIX innervation of the Eustachian tube tube may result in transmission of the virus to the brainsem after original infection of the external acoustic meatus and thence middle ear and Eustachian tube. It is possible that this may be the sole route of infection especially in case of occlusion of the auditory tube. The current prophylactic measures have ignored this route of infection, advising masks that cover the nose and the mouth, leaving the ear unprotected. Despite my early alerting of the relevant health agencies, my advice has not been heeded.

Viral infections of CNIX give rise to well known diseases and may occur concurrently with infections of other cranial nerves [15].

CNX vagus nerve

The vagus nerve is not only a long, wandering nerve in the cervical, thoracic, and abdominal areas, it also carries a host of fiber types, motor, autonomic, viscerosensory, chemosensory, and somatosensory.

The motor fibers of the vagus nerve originate in the *nucleus ambiguus* and innervate the pharynx, larynx and palate. Injury or compromise of any kind in these fibers will result in paralysis of pharyngeal muscles, the gag reflex, and partial or total paralysis of laryngeal muscles. Paralysis of the *vocal cords* will result in changes in vocalization, difficulty in breathing or total inability to breath and death.

The vagal fibers to the intrinsic muscles of the larynx first join CNXI, spinal accessory nerve, rejoin CNX and descend into the thoracic cavity where they split off as *recurrent laryngeal nerve* which loops around the aortic arch and ascends along the trachea to innervate the larynx as i*nferior laryngeal nerve.*

In the early stages of viral infection the pharynx is one

of the first areas affected. This is manifested in the reported persistent dry cough. I is very likely that in a mater of a few days the virus reaches the brainstem via retrograde axonal transport to nucleus ambiguus.

Nucleus solitarius may be infected by axonal transport of the virus:in viscerosensory fibers from the pharynx and larynx. This may account for the observed loss of taste.

This route of virus infection of brainstem nuclei is probably the best candidate for the initial infection. Virus transport from the nose via CNI would take more time not only because of greater distance but also the number of intervening synapses.

CNX is also the great highway of autonomic parasympatheric innervation of the heart, lungs and intestines. We need to remind ourselves that the *autonomic nervous system* is motor for smooth muscle, cardiac muscle, and glands. Compromise of this component of the vagus nerve because of trauma, infection or pharmacological interventions results in dramatic effects on cardiovascular, secretory and motor responses of intrinsic pulmonary muscles.

The observed pneumonia-like phase in some COVID-19 patients very likely involves the vagus nerve. Anterograde axonal transport to the lungs and heart, although possible, would be delayed, as the direct transport of the virus via the trachea and possibly *retropharyngeal space* is the most likely route. However, the development of serious pulmonary disease in some patients must be partly the result of compromised function of vagal components, and not solely of immunologic nature. As the response of pulmonary muscles is not only depended on the traditional cholinergic and adrenergic effects, but it also involves nitric oxide (NO) and vasoactive intestinal polypeptide (VIP), no easy suggestions can be made as to the mode of vagal effects on cardio pulmonary disease. A compromised vagal cholinergic pathway would result to disturbances in the interaction of vagus and immune system.

Viral infections of CNX give rise to well known diseases and may occur concurrently with infections of other cranial nerves [16].

{ 16 }

CNXI spinal accessory nerve

The accessory part of CNXI (accessory to vagus) is of possible significance in COVID-19 disease as its fibers stem from *nucleus ambiguous* and innervate the intrinsic muscles of the larynx. The clinical manifestation of damage to these fibers is discussed in the vagus nerve section above.

Viral infections of CNXI give rise to well known diseases and may occur concurrently with infections of other cranial nerves [16].

{ 17 }

CNXII hypoglossal nerve

The hypoglossal nerve is a motor nerve that innervates the muscles of the tongue. Despite their location, these muscles are not branchiomeric, they are somatic. Thus the hypoglossal nerve may be considered a spinal nerve. The location of the hypoglossal nucleus in the medulla as well as the fact that this nerve contains fibers of cervical spinal nerves supports such a proposition.

Viral infection of the tongue has been shown to be transported retrogradely to the CNXII nucleus [16].

Epilogue

Variations in the progression of COVID-19 as well as the serious pulmonary disease in a small percentage of patients, may point to CNS nerve routes and mechanisms, in addition to systemic ones. The extensive, omnipresent nervous system network and the transport mechanisms it employs needs to be considered along with molecular, pharmacological interventions.

Progression of the disease is determined by an unpredictable engagement of variables in time due to spatiotemporal constraints. This non-linear engagement demands that we keep in mind a picture of pseudo quantal causative contributions in time.

The most dramatic and gravest component of COVID-19 is pulmonary disease. Understanding the anatomy and physiology of the nervous system is crucial in planning preventive strategies as well as devising therapeutic interventions.

{ 19 }

References

1. Li YC, Bai WZ, Hashikawa T. The neuroinvasive potential of SARS-CoV2 may play a role in the respiratory failure of COVID-19 patients [published online ahead of print, 2020 Feb 27]. *J Med Virol.* 2020;10.1002/jmv.25728. doi:10.1002/jmv.25728

2. Shaobo Shi, MD; Mu Qin, MD; Bo Shen, MD; et al. Association of Cardiac Injury With Mortality in Hospitalized Patients With COVID-19 in Wuhan, China. AMA Cardiol. Published online March 25, 2020. doi:10.1001/jamacardio.2020.0950

3. Dubé M, Le Coupanec A, Wong AHM, Rini JM, Desforges M, Talbot PJ. Axonal Transport Enables Neuron-to-Neuron Propagation of Human Coronavirus OC43. *J Virol.* 2018;92(17):e00404-18. Published 2018 Aug 16. doi:10.1128/JVI.00404-18

4. van Riel D, Verdijk R, Kuiken T. The olfactory nerve: a shortcut for influenza and other viral diseases into the central nervous system. *J Pathol.* 2015;235(2):277-287. doi:10.1002/path.446

5. Kahloun R, Abroug N, Ksiaa I, et al. Infectious optic neuropathies: a clinical update. *Eye Brain.* 2015;7:59-81. Published 2015 Sep 28. doi:10.2147/EB.S69173

6. Wei H, Yin H, Huang M, Guo Z. The 2019 novel coronavirus pneumonia with onset of oculomotor nerve palsy: a case study. *J Neurol.* 2020;267(5):1550-1553. doi:10.1007/s00415-020-09773-9

7. Park KC, Yoon SS, Yoon JE, Rhee HY. A case of herpes zoster ophthalmicus with isolated trochlear nerve involvement. *J Clin Neurol.* 2011;7(1):47-49. doi:10.3988/jcn.2011.7.1.47

8. Folan-Curran J, Hickey K, Monkhouse WS. Innervation of the rat external auditory meatus: a retrograde tracing study. *Somatosens Mot Res.* 1994;11(1):65-68. doi:10.3109/08990229409028858

9. Ptaszyńska-Sarosiek I, Dunaj J, Zajkowska A, et al. Postmortem detection of six human herpesviruses (HSV-1, HSV-2, VZV, EBV, CMV, HHV-6) in trigeminal and facial nerve ganglia by PCR. *PeerJ.* 2019;6:e6095. Published 2019 Jan 9. doi:10.7717/peerj.6095

10. Cohen HA, Nussinovitch M, Ashkenazi A, Straussberg R, Kaushansky A. Benign abducens nerve palsy of childhood. *Pediatr Neurol.* 1993;9(5):394-395. doi:10.1016/0887-8994(93)90110-x

11. Greco F, Garozzo R, Sorge G. Isolated abducens nerve palsy complicating cytomegalovirus infection. *Pediatr Neurol.* 2006;35(3):229-230. doi:10.1016/j.pediatrneurol.2006.03.008

12. E.G. Antzoulatos, A.C. Kalyva, C.F. Flaherty, and M.M. Nikoletseas. Dishabituation of the Branchial Defensive Reflex in Goldfish, Carassius auratus, in Relation to Sensitization and Different Levels of Prior Habituation.. Soc. Neurosci. Abstr., Vol 23, Part 2, p.1620, 1997

13. Davis LE. Experimental viral infections of the facial nerve and geniculate ganglion. *Ann Neurol.* 1981;9(2):120-125. doi:10.1002/ana.410090204

14. Cohen BE, Durstenfeld A, Roehm PC. Viral causes of hearing loss: a review for hearing health professionals. *Trends Hear.* 2014;18:2331216514541361. Published 2014 Jul 29. doi:10.1177/2331216514541361

15. Finsterer J, Grisold W. Disorders of the lower cranial nerves. *J Neurosci Rural Pract.* 2015;6(3):377-391. doi:10.4103/0976-3147.158768

16. Openshaw H, Ellis WG. Herpes simplex virus infection of motor neurons: hypoglossal model. *Infect Immun.* 1983;42(1):409-413

{ 20 }

General bibliography

Bordoni B, Purgol S, Bizzarri A, Modica M, Morabito B. The Influence of Breathing on the Central Nervous System. *Cureus*. 2018;10(6):e2724. Published 2018 Jun 1. doi:10.7759/cureus.2724

Li YC, Bai WZ, Hashikawa T. The neuroinvasive potential of SARS-CoV2 may play a role in the respiratory failure of COVID-19 patients [published online ahead of print, 2020 Feb 27]. *J Med Virol*. 2020;10.1002/jmv.25728. doi:10.1002/jmv.25728

Nikoletseas, Michael M. Behavioral and Neural Plasticity , 2010. ISBN 10: 1453789456 ISBN 13: 9781453789452

Nikoletseas, Michael M. Cranial Nerves for Medical Students: with clinical correlations,

2010. ISBN-10: 1453812946; ISBN-13: 978-1453812945

Nikoletseas, Michael . Retropharyngeal infection in Covid-19 patient cardiac injury, March 2020.

DOI: 10.13140/RG.2.2.17870.00328

Mathieu Dubé, Alain Le Coupanec, Alan H. M. Wong,

James M. Rini, Marc Desforges, Pierre J. Talbot. Michael S. Diamond, Editor. Axonal Transport Enables Neuron-to-Neuron Propagation of Human Coronavirus OC43

DOI: 10.1128/JVI.00404-18

Ikeda, K., Kawakami, K., Onimaru, H. et al. The respiratory control mechanisms in the brainstem and spinal cord: integrative views of the neuroanatomy and neurophysiology. J Physiol Sci 67, 45–62 (2017). https://doi.org/10.1007/s12576-016-0475-y

Charles S. Bryan, MD; Barry G. King Jr., MD; Richard E. Bryant, MD. Retropharyngeal Infection in Adults. Arch Intern Med. 1974;134(1):127-130. doi:10.1001/archinte.1974.00320190129020

Prof Francois-Xavier Lescure, MD, Prof Lila Bouadma, MD, Duc Nguyen, MD, Marion Parisey, MD, Paul-Henri Wicky, MD, Sylvie Behillil, PharmD, et al.. Clinical and virological data of the first cases of COVID-19 in Europe: a case series

DOI:https://doi.org/10.1016/S1473-3099(20)30200-0

The Lancet https://www.thelancet.com/journals/laninf/article/PIIS1473-3099(20)30200-0/fulltext

Yeshun Wu,a,b,1 Xiaolin Xu,c,1 Zijun Chen,b Jiahao Duan,b Kenji Hashimoto,d Ling Yang,b Cunming Liu,a,? and Chun Yanga,?

Nervous system involvement after infection with COVID-19 and other coronaviruses. Brain Behav Immun. 2020 Mar 30

doi: 10.1016/j.bbi.2020.03.031 [Epub ahead of print]
PMCID: PMC7146689, PMID: 32240762

Charles S. Bryan, MD; Barry G. King Jr., MD; Richard E. Bryant, MD. Retropharyngeal Infection in Adults. Arch Intern Med. 1974;134(1):127-130. doi:10.1001/archinte.1974.00320190129020

Shaobo Shi, MD; Mu Qin, MD; Bo Shen, MD; et al. Association of Cardiac Injury With Mortality in Hospitalized Patients With COVID-19 in Wuhan, China. AMA Cardiol. Published online March 25, 2020. doi:10.1001/jamacardio.2020.0950

Russell Thomas Woodburne, William E. Burkel. Essentials of Human Anatomy. Oxford University Press, 1994

Steven D. Waldman MD, JD, Retropharyngeal Abscess, I n Atlas of Common Pain Syndromes (Fourth Edition), Elsevier, 2019

Jeffrey C. Kwong, M.D., Kevin L. Schwartz, M.D., Michael A. Campitelli, M.P.H., Hannah Chung, M.P.H., Natasha S. Crowcroft, M.D., Timothy Karnauchow, Ph.D., Kevin Katz, M.D., Dennis T. Ko, M.D., Allison J. McGeer, M.D., Dayre McNally, M.D., Ph.D., David C. Richardson, M.D., Laura C. Rosella, Ph.D., M.H.Sc., Andrew Simor, M.D., Marek Smieja, M.D., Ph.D., George Zahariadis, M.D., and Jonathan B. Gubbay, M.B., B.S., M.Med.Sc. et al. Acute Myocardial Infarction after Laboratory-Confirmed Influenza Infection. N Engl J Med 2018; 378:345-353

DOI: 10.1056/NEJMoa1702090

Ian M. Balfour-Lynn BSc, MD, MBBS, FRCP, FRCPCH, FRCS (Ed), DHMSA, Jane C. Davies MB, ChB, MRCP, MRCPCH, MD, in Kendig & Chernick's Disorders of the Respiratory Tract in Children (Eighth Edition), 2012

Jeong Hee Shin, MD, Se In Sung, MD, Jin Kyu Kim, MD, Ji Mi Jung, MD, Eun Sun Kim, MD, Soo Han Choi, MD, Yae Jean Kim, MD, Kang Mo Ahn, MD, Yun Sil Chang, MD, and Won Soon Park, MD. Retropharyngeal abscess coinfected with Staphylococcus aureus and Mycobacterium tuberculosis after rhinoviral infection in a 1-month-old infant. Korean J Pediatr. 2013 Feb; 56(2): 86–89.

Marc Tebruegge, Nigel Curtis, in Principles and Practice of Pediatric Infectious Diseases (Fifth Edition), 2018

Hoang, JK; Branstetter BF, 4th; Eastwood, JD; Glastonbury, CM (April 2011). "Multiplanar CT and MRI of collections in the retropharyngeal space: is it an abscess?". AJR. American Journal of Roentgenology. 196 (4): W426-32. doi:10.2214/AJR.10.5116. PMID 21427307

Michael Nikoletseas. Retropharyngeal infection in Covid-19 patient cardiac injury.
DOI: 10.13140/RG.2.2.17870.00328
https://www.researchgate.net/publication/340246631_Retropharyngeal_infection_in_Covid-19_patient_cardiac_injury?channel=doi&linkId=5e7ea7dc299bf1a91b827e10&showFulltext=true

R. D. Mooney, M. M. Nikoletseas, S. A. Ruiz, and R. W. Rhoades. Receptive-field properties and morphological characteristics of the superior collicular neurons that project to the lateral posterior and dorsal lateral geniculate nuclei in the hamster. Journal of Neurophysiology 59 (5), 1333-1351
https://doi.org/10.1152/jn.1988.59.5.1333

Nikoletseas, Michael. Urgent revision of prophylactic measures against COVID-19.

DOI: 10.13140/RG.2.2.15227.26407

https://www.researchgate.net/publication/
339943615_URGENT_REVISION_OF_PROPHYLAC-
TIC_MEASURES_AGAINST_COVID-19?

channel=doi&linkId=5e6e78d4458515e5557fa836&show-
Fulltext=true

Nikoletseas, Michael. The significance of observed loss of taste in COVID-19.

DOI : 10.13140/RG.2.2.33051.41766/1 htps://www.re-searchgate.net/publication/340163920_The_signifi-cance_of_observed_loss_of_taste_in_COVID-19, March 2020

Nikoletseas, Michael. The significance of observed anosmia in COVID-19.

DOI: 10.13140/RG.2.2.32291.20007/1 htps://www.re-searchgate.net/publication/340117636_The_signifi-cance_of_observed_anosmia_in_COVID-19
?channel=doi&linkId=5e7a02c292851c3091393179&show-
Fulltext=true

Wani A, Rehman A, Lateef S, Malik R, Ahmed A, Ahmad W, et al. Traumatic tympanic membrane perforation:An overview. Indian J Otol. 2016;22(2):100–104

Matthew L Howard, MD, JD; Chief Editor: Arlen D Meyers, MD, MBA more... What is the medical treatment for tympanic membrane perforation (TMP)?

https://www.medscape.com/answers/858684-63655/
what-is-the-medical-treatment-for-tympanicmembrane-
perforation-tmp

Arwa Kurabi, Kwang K. Pak, Marlen Bernhardt, Andrew Baird & Allen F. Ryan. Mechanism of Active Transport through the Tympanic Membrane to the Middle Ear. Scientific Reports volume 6, Article number: 22663 (2016)

Varicella zoster virus infection of the pharynx and larynx with multiple cranial neuropathies.

Lin YY, Kao CH, Wang CH

Laryngoscope. 2011 Aug; 121(8):1627-30

Cohen BE, Durstenfeld A, Roehm PC. Viral causes of hearing loss: a review for hearing health professionals. *Trends Hear*. 2014;18:2331216514541361. Published 2014 Jul 29. doi:10.1177/2331216514541361

Qingshan Teng, Thais Federici, Nicholas M.Boulis. Viral Vector Axonal Uptake and Retrograde Transport: Mechanisms and Applications, in Gene Therapy of the Central Nervous System, Academic Press, 2006, pages 253-271

About the author

Dr. Michael Nikoletseas did his undergraduate work at Roosevelt University in Psychology and Biology (B.A. With Honors), his graduate work in Psychobiology at Rutgers University (M.S., Ph.D.), and his post-doctoral training in Medical Anatomy at the Medical College of Pennsylvania, and University of Medicine and Dentistry of New Jersey. He has taught Anatomy at the University of Wisconsin Medical School in Madison, and other US institutions. In addition to his research publications in neuroanatomy and neurophysiology he has written books in Medicine, Neuroscience and Mathematics.

Lightning Source UK Ltd.
Milton Keynes UK
UKHW021055010620
364249UK00004B/602